Withdrawn

SURVIVAL
FIRST AID

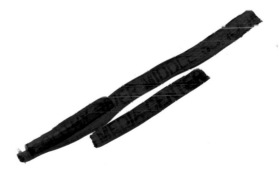

ELITE FORCES SURVIVAL GUIDE SERIES

Elite Survival
Survive in the Desert with the French Foreign Legion
Survive in the Arctic with the Royal Marine Commandos
Survive in the Mountains with the U.S. Rangers and Army
  Mountain Division
Survive in the Jungle with the Special Forces "Green Berets"
Survive in the Wilderness with the Canadian and Australian
  Special Forces
Survive at Sea with the U.S. Navy SEALs
Training to Fight with the Parachute Regiment
The World's Best Soldiers

Elite Operations and Training
Escape and Evasion
Surviving Captivity with the U.S. Air Force
Hostage Rescue with the SAS
How to Pass Elite Forces Selection
Learning Mental Endurance with the U.S. Marines

Special Forces Survival Guidebooks
Survival Equipment
Navigation and Signaling
Surviving Natural Disasters
Using Ropes and Knots
Survival First Aid
Trapping, Fishing, and Plant Food
Urban Survival Techniques

SURVIVAL
FIRST AID

PATRICK WILSON

Introduction by Colonel John T. Carney. Jr., USAF–Ret.
President, Special Operations Warrior Foundation

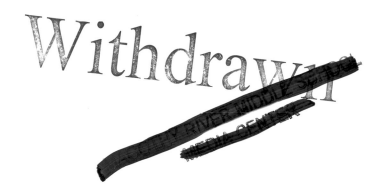

MASON CREST PUBLISHERS

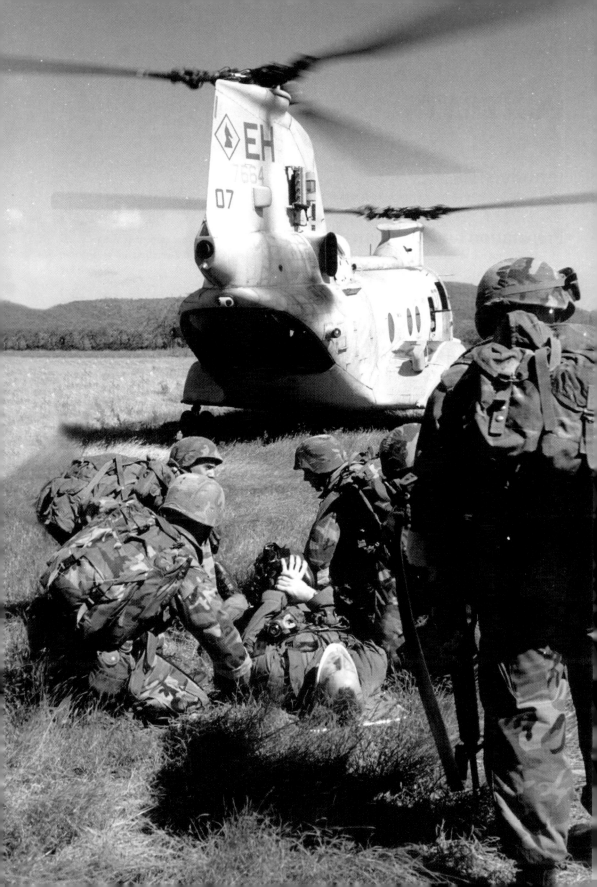

INTRODUCTION

Elite forces are the tip of Freedom's spear. These small, special units are universally the first to engage, whether on reconnaissance missions into denied territory for larger, conventional forces or in direct action, surgical operations, preemptive strikes, retaliatory action, and hostage rescues. They lead the way in today's war on terrorism, the war on drugs, the war on transnational unrest, and in humanitarian operations as well as nation building. When large scale warfare erupts, they offer theater commanders a wide variety of unique, unconventional options.

Most such units are regionally oriented, acclimated to the culture and conversant in the languages of the areas where they operate. Since they deploy to those areas regularly, often for combined training exercises with indigenous forces, these elite units also serve as peacetime "global scouts" and "diplomacy multipliers," a beacon of hope for the democratic aspirations of oppressed peoples all over the globe.

Elite forces are truly "quiet professionals": their actions speak louder than words. They are self-motivated, self-confident, versatile, seasoned, mature individuals who rely on teamwork more than daring-do. Unfortunately, theirs is dangerous work. Since "Desert One"—the 1980 attempt to rescue hostages from the U.S. embassy in Tehran, for instance—American special operations forces have suffered casualties in real world operations at close to fifteen times the rate of U.S. conventional forces. By the very nature of the challenges which face special operations forces, training for these elite units has proven even more hazardous.

Thus it's with special pride that I join you in saluting the brave men and women who volunteer to serve in and support these magnificent units and who face such difficult challenges ahead.

Colonel John T. Carney, Jr., USAF–Ret.
President, Special Operations Warrior Foundation

U.S. Army soldiers attend to a "patient" during a simulated casualty exercise in 1998. All elite troops are trained in first-aid techniques.

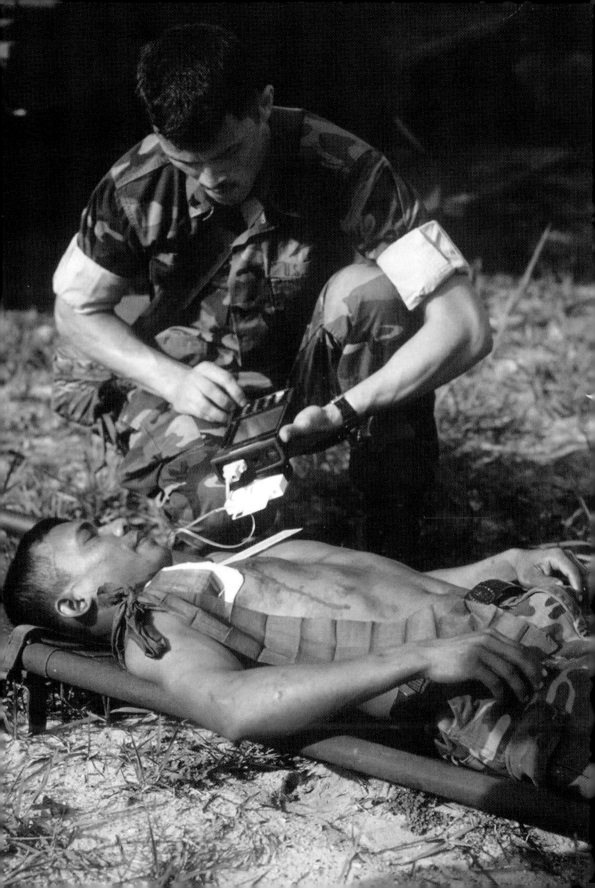

DECIDING ON A COURSE
OF ACTION

Troops are thoroughly trained in dealing with an emergency situation since it can be very shocking. Their first response should be to take deep breaths and then begin to assess the situation calmly, however traumatic it might appear. They then follow this step-by-step procedure.

First, it is important to see if there are any new dangers present and establish who has been injured. In any accident situation, where there may be injured people, always check for dangers to yourself before approaching victims. Such dangers include electric cables, fires, gas pipes, falling debris, dangerous structures, or wreckage. If there are two or more persons present, one is put in charge to avoid confusion. They then follow the DATE system:

- **Diagnosis**—working out quickly what the patient's illness or injury is.
- Assessment—working out the best form of first-aid treatment.
- Treatment—giving treatment to the injured person.
- Evacuation—making sure that the patient is taken to a proper medical center or doctor if he or she is very ill or badly injured.

This soldier, taking part in a training exercise at Fort Polk, Louisiana, in 2001 is taught to identify medical emergencies quickly. Once the problem is identified, he must then take appropriate action.

airway. This may stop the person from breathing. Other objects such as food may also be lodged there.

If this has happened, a soldier will open the casualty's mouth and inspect for any blockages first. The mouth is then cleared of any obvious blood or vomit. Once this is done, the tongue is eased forward to open the airway. To keep the airway open, the casualty's head is moved.

One hand is put on the casualty's forehead, and two fingers from the other hand are placed under the point of the chin. The victim's head is gently tilted backward, moving very slowly and carefully in case there are any spinal or neck injuries.

This action will open the airway enough for the patient to breathe. The patient is placed in the **recovery position** to make it easier to breathe.

Breathing

Once the airway has been cleared (this takes only a few seconds), the

RAPID ASSESSMENT WITH THE SPECIAL FORCES

A rapid assessment of any first-aid situation is vital. Knowing who to treat first can save lives. These are the priorities, as laid down by the Special Forces, for dealing with injuries in an emergency situation: restore and maintain breathing and heartbeat, stop bleeding, protect wounds and burns, deal with bone fractures, and treat shock.

casualty's breathing is checked. This is done by bending down and placing a cheek right next to the casualty's mouth and nose. Eyes should be kept on the casualty's chest. This will give you three opportunities to detect lack of breathing—you should feel the casualty's breath on your cheek, hear it, and also see the rise and fall of the chest. If all these signs

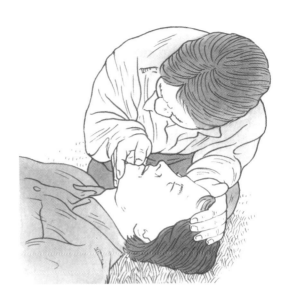

A first-aider checks this casualty's breathing for signs of life by placing his hand in front of the nose and mouth.

are absent for over 10 seconds, then it is necessary to begin giving **resuscitation**.

Circulation

The basic principle here is to check for any major sources of blood or fluid loss, and to monitor the heartbeat. Checking for blood loss involves finding any source of heavy bleeding and stemming the flow using the most appropriate technique. In a cold climate, a soldier must check all areas of the body. Heavy, layered waterproof clothing can often hide areas of bleeding.

Troops check for the **pulse** in one of two places. The first is the artery in the wrist. A soldier places three fingers (never the thumb: this has a pulse of its own, which may confuse matters) over the

- Arms and hands—troops, like the Special Forces, are instructed to look for any breakages or swellings. They are taught to examine fingernails for any blueness. This tends to indicate circulation or breathing disorders. The casualty is asked if they feel any strange sensations, such as numbness or pins and needles. This helps judge any nerve or spinal damage. One test is to ask the casualty to squeeze your two forefingers. If the strength of grip is not the same, this may indicate a stroke or physical damage to the limb.
- Legs and feet—if the casualty is still able to walk, trained members

SKIN COLORATION

The following skin colors give elite troops clues as to what is wrong with the casualty:

- Blue or blue/gray: especially if prominent in the lips and fingernails, may indicate that the patient is lacking oxygen. This may be caused by disrupted breathing, a heart attack, or other cardiac problems. If the person is unconscious, it might indicate malaria.
- Darkened skin: can be a symptom of starvation.
- Pale skin: if combined with cool, moist texture, suggests shock. Skin lightening can also occur with a lack of protein or hypothermia.
- Red skin: may indicate poisoning; fever; heatstroke; sunburn.

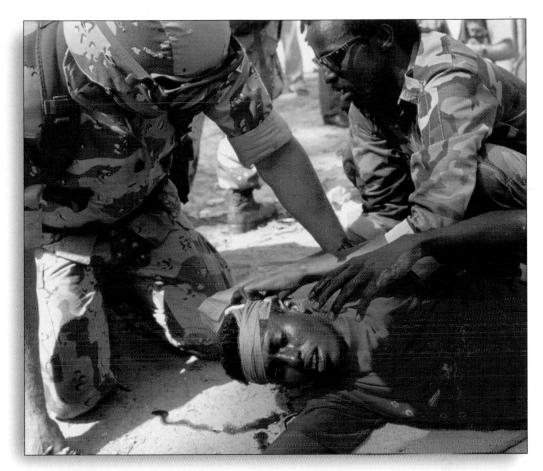

A casualty with a head injury sustained during riots in Haiti in 1994 is attended to by U.S. Marine soldiers Correct bandaging is essential to prevent infections in this case.

of an elite force will ask the person to walk in a straight line so that they can check his balance. If the victims are conscious and lying down, they are told to pull and push their feet backward and forward against the resistance of a soldier's hands. Any differences between the strength levels of the two limbs may indicate nerve or spinal damage. Elite troops check nerve responses by scratching the soles of the patient's feet to test the tickle response.

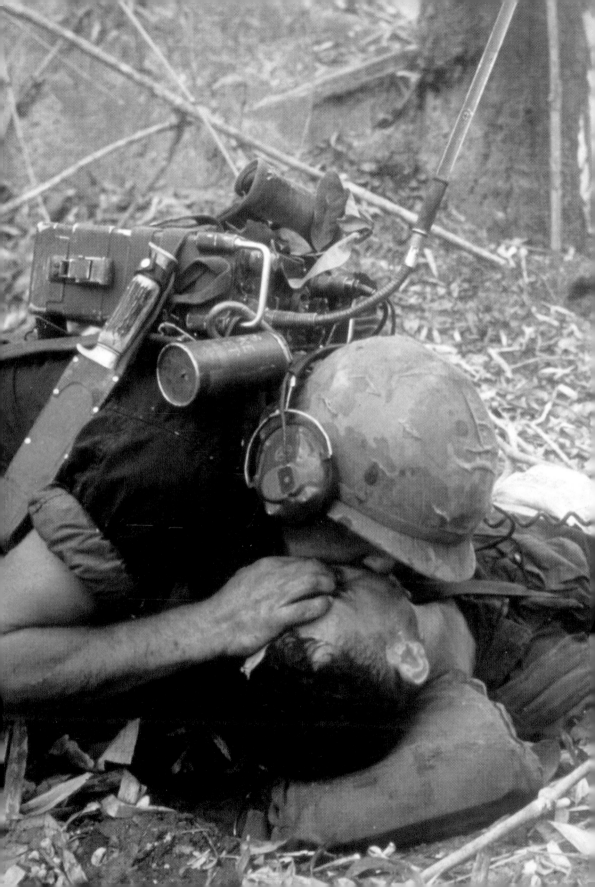

BREATHING AND CIRCULATION

Few first-aid situations are more serious than when casualties' hearts stop pumping or when they are unable to breathe. If left untreated, brain death can occur within five minutes. Death can follow soon after, and there is nothing any member of the elite forces can do in such a situation.

Stoppage of the heart can have a variety of causes. A heart attack, major blood loss, and **hypothermia** are among the major causes likely to be encountered by elite troops in a survival situation. Absence of pulse and the absence of breathing are the major signs that this has happened.

Soldiers need to be cautious because, in cold conditions especially, an injured person's pulse and circulation can become very difficult to detect. This is because the cold slows down the system. It is important to be very sure that the person's heart really has stopped before taking emergency action.

Artificial respiration

This is the practice of externally supplying casualties with enough air in order to make sure they have enough oxygen in the blood. The most common and well-known artificial method is known as mouth-to-mouth **respiration**. This is where the first-aider breathes

Vietnam War, 1962. A medic gives CPR (cardiopulmonary resuscitation) in an attempt to get this wounded soldier breathing again.

into the casualty's mouth in order to get air into the lungs. The technique is as follows:

Step 1: The casualty's head is tilted back by placing one hand on the forehead and lifting under the point of the chin with the two forefingers of the other hand. The head should not be moved if there are any spinal injuries. The head tilt lifts the tongue away from the entrance to the windpipe and ensures the free passage of air down to the lungs.

Step 2: The casualty's nostrils are then pinched, while the first-aider's mouth is sealed around the casualty's mouth. The first-aider then blows. This should make the patient's chest rise. Once the first-aider's mouth is removed, the chest muscles will force the air out of the lungs. The process is then repeated until the casualty begins to breathe alone again. The pattern should be six immediate breaths as fast as possible, before setting up a rhythm of about 12 cycles a minute.

A   B

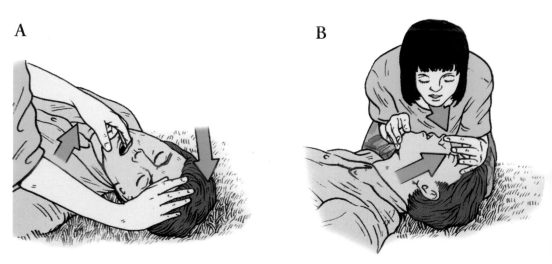

A step-by-step guide to mouth-to-mouth resuscitation. (A) Clear the airway of blockages. (B) Tilt the victim's head backward, raise their

Cardiac massage

This is a technique used by elite troops, like the U.S. Marines and French Foreign Legion, to pump a casualty's blood if there is no effective heartbeat. By pressing down on the breastbone, which is positioned directly above the heart, blood is squeezed out of the heart. Once the pressure is released, blood flows back in. The technique is as follows:

Step 1: After kneeling next to the casualty, a finger should be run up one of the lowest ribs until it meets the breastbone. The heel of the first-aider's hand should be placed about one finger's width above this point, then he or she brings the other hand on top and interlocks the fingers.

Step 2: Following this, the first-aider leans right over the casualty with the arms straight and presses the breastbone down by about one and a half to two inches (3–5 cm). The first-aider then releases the pressure but keeps the hands ready on the spot and follows with

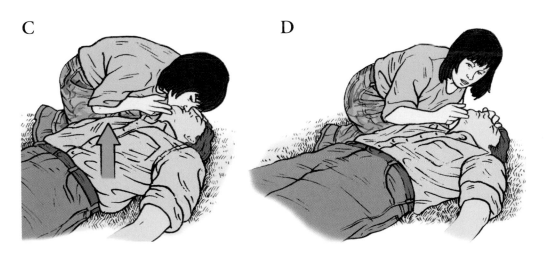

chin, and pinch their nose. **(C)** Take a deep breath and blow air into their mouth. **(D)** Stop blowing when the victim's chest expands.

another **compression**. The compressions are maintained at a rate of about 100 pushes a minute. This is very tiring.

A member of the elite forces will not give up with the **cardiac** massage procedure. They will continue for at least an hour if necessary. Because cardiac massage can be tiring, it is important to take turns if there is a group.

Cardiopulmonary resuscitation (CPR)

This is where both cardiac massage and mouth-to-mouth resuscitation are used. It is an important technique because when the patient's heart stops, so does breathing.

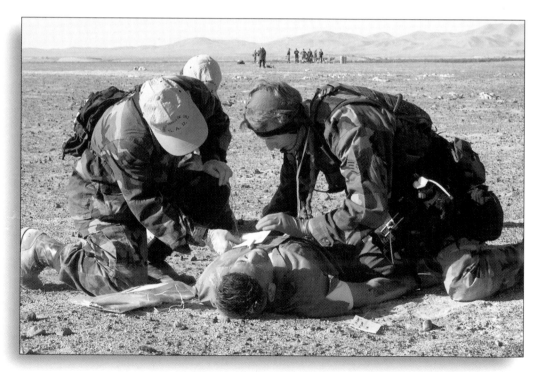

Soldiers from the Chilean Air Force assess a patient's condition before giving CPR in the Atacama Desert, September 2000.

CPR can save a patient who would otherwise die. It is very important. These are the instructions given to Canadian Special Forces troops in training:

- Check for consciousness.
- Establish an open airway.
- Look, listen, and feel for breathing.
- Give four rapid breaths.
- Check for pulse (while you look, listen, and feel for breaths).
- Locate the compression spot.
- Form proper hand position.
- Begin compressions: set of 15 compressions, then…
- Two quick breaths after each set of 15 compressions.
- After four complete sets of 15 compressions, two breaths, check for at least five seconds for pulse and breathing.
- If there are no signs, continue for as long as is necessary.

Respiratory accidents
Near-drowning
If water is nearby, drowning is a constant danger. It can happen very quickly. In cold water, it is possible for a person to lose consciousness in seconds. A further danger, witnessed in about 15 percent of drownings, is that the throat goes into **spasm** and closes completely.

Troops know that treatment needs to be quick and decisive. Once the person has been rescued, carry him from the water with the head lower than the rest of the body to help get the water from the stomach. On the bank, the casualty should be put on his back.

It is important not to try to pump out water out of his lungs. However, the casualty should have his breathing and pulse checked in the normal way. Bear in mind, however, that it is harder to find the pulse and to check breathing if a person has been in cold water.

If the casualty is definitely not breathing and has no pulse, then CPR should be performed on him. Once breathing is restored, the person should be moved into the recovery position. This is

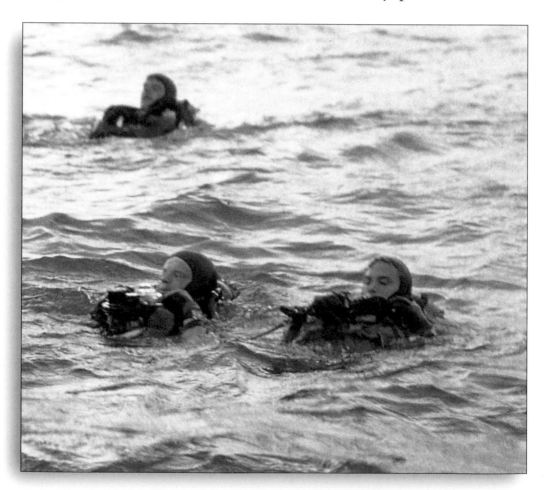

U.S. Navy SEALs are highly experienced swimmers. They undergo a strict training program, which makes it unlikely they would ever drown.

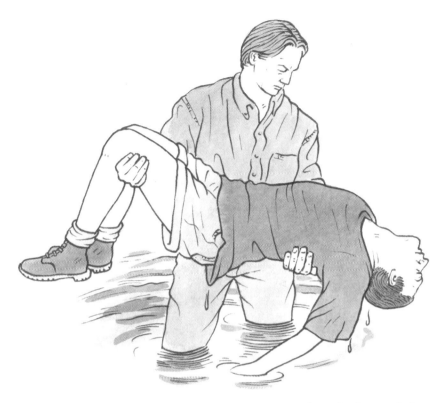

The "head back" position is recommended for victims of drowning because it makes it easier for water to flow back out of the lungs.

not the end of the treatment. The person is wet and shocked and may be susceptible to hypothermia. The casualty is therefore given dry clothing and placed in a position sheltered from the wind.

Choking

People suffering from blocked airways are unable to breathe and, unless they are already unconscious, will be very distressed and red-faced. They will probably be violently pointing to or clutching their throats. If they are found unconscious, they will have a gray blue complexion, the color that indicates a person is suffering from a lack of oxygen.

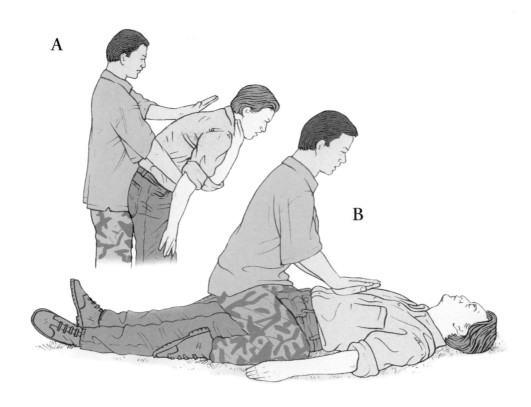

The two-stage technique used to relieve a blockage from a patient who is choking, whether conscious (A) or unconscious (B).

Note: If people are coughing, no matter how violently, then a soldier knows they are not choking. Their bodies are just naturally trying to get rid of the blockage.

The most common form of blockage is food, but other causes of choking can be from the tongue or from a throat swelling caused by an allergic reaction. If it is a blockage and the person is conscious, he should be encouraged to cough. If this does not clear the blockage, they should be bent forward and given five sharp slaps between the shoulder blades. If the obstruction has still not come forward, the first-aider should perform the Heimlich maneuver.

THE HEIMLICH MANEUVER

This antichoking method, named after Henry J. Heimlich, the man who first invented it, is performed by elite troops around the world. It is the most reliable means of freeing a blockage in a patient's throat during an emergency situation.

- Stand behind the casualty and wrap your arms around her waist.
- Make a fist and place it just beneath the casualty's breastbone with thumb against the chest. Grip this fist with your other hand.
- Pull your fist sharply in and up. Repeat three times, then check the mouth.

This action forces air in the lungs up the windpipe. The air pushes the obstacle out like a cork from a bottle.

Smoke and fumes inhalation

In outdoor survival situations, where there is plenty of fresh air, the dangers of breathing in smoke or fumes are small. However, there are exceptions such as:

- Carbon monoxide—the main sources of carbon monoxide are faulty gas or paraffin heaters, stoves used in tents, and fire smoke. Carbon monoxide deprives the body of oxygen. It is very dangerous and has no odor. **Symptoms** include fatigue, confusion, and even aggression. This leads to breathing failure and unconsciousness. Death can occur.

• Smoke—any sort of smoke reduces the levels of oxygen in the air and can sometimes make breathing impossible. It is unlikely members of one of the elite forces would suffer this, unless they found themselves unexpectedly engulfed in a forest fire or in a burning building.

It is important that elite rescuers do not put themselves in danger from the gas, fumes, or smoke. If they are not in immediate danger, rescue teams should pull the casualty out of the danger area and into fresh air. If there is little fresh air available, rescuers should cover their mouths with light material. They should then follow the standard procedure used to check breathing, consciousness, and circulation. Rescuers should note that mouth-to-mouth rescusitation might well be required.

A Special Air Service (SAS) soldier in a counter-revolutionary warfare outfit. He wears a gas mask at all times.

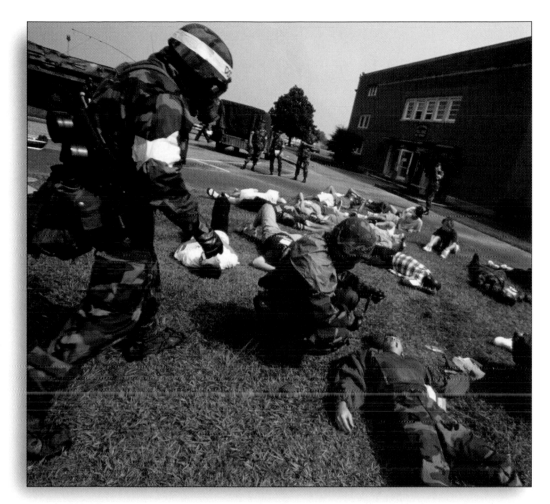

U.S. Marines take part in a decontamination training exercise in North Carolina. Even today, chemical warfare remains a reality of battle.

Shock

This occurs when there is not enough blood circulating in the body of the patient. It can be caused by bleeding, breaking bones, and loss of fluids through sweating, vomiting, and diarrhea. Shock is a likely diagnosis if a person has pale, cold, and clammy skin, a fast and weak pulse, and fast and shallow breathing.

To treat this, soldiers check to see the airway is open. Any bone breakages will be treated. The patient should be kept warm and still. Any rough handling of a casualty suffering from shock is very dangerous and therefore forbidden.

Shock can be a killer. In the wild, you must recognize the symptoms and treat them. These are the guidelines the U.S. Army gives to troops:

- If conscious, place the patient on a level surface, and slightly raise the legs. This will help to generate blood flow to the core organs and the head.
- If unconscious, place the patient on the side with the head turned to one side to prevent choking.
- Once the patient is in shock position, do not move.
- Keep the patient warm. Heat loss and hypothermia will

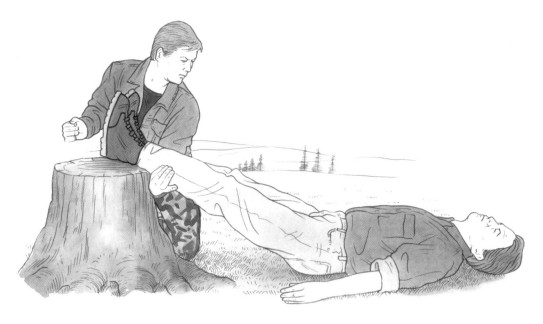

One of the best treatments for shock is to increase the blood supply to the patient's vital organs. This can be done by raising the legs.

accelerate shock. You should also place something (a blanket, for instance) between the patient and the cold ground.

- If the patient is wet, remove all wet clothing as quickly as possible and replace with dry items.
- Cover the patient with clothing, tree boughs, and shelter him or her from the weather.
- Use hot liquids, food, or body heat to provide warmth.
- Only give patients liquids or foods if they are conscious, and do not give them if the patients have **abdominal** wounds.
- Let the patient rest for at least 24 hours.

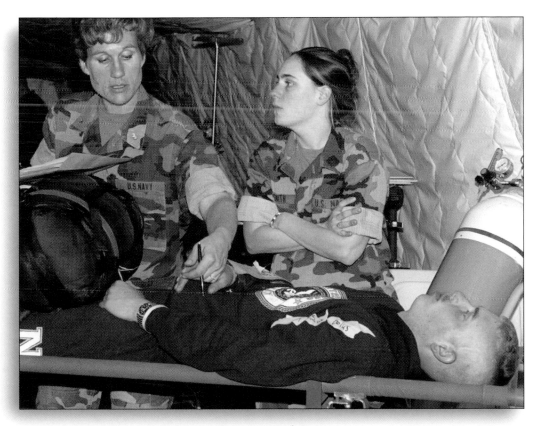

Medical training at Camp Lejeune, North Carolina. Training should be so intense that treatment becomes second nature.

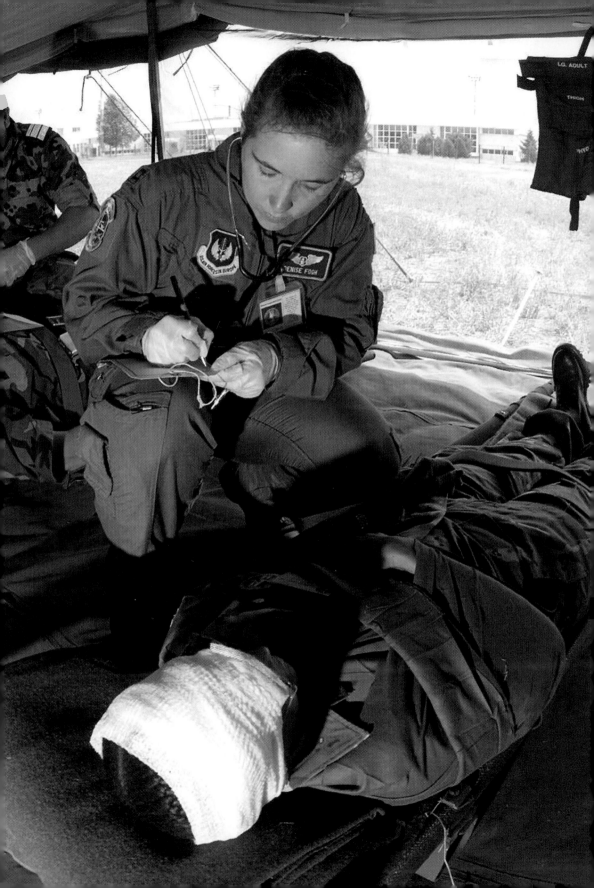

WOUNDS, BLEEDING, AND BURNS

Wounds and blood loss are the most common forms of injury for elite troops because they spend much of their time in battle against enemy soldiers. There are three main types of bleeding, which vary in their degree of seriousness.

Arterial bleeding is blood in the arteries that is under high pressure. If an artery is cut, the victim is in danger of a fatal loss of blood, and could die within minutes. Arterial blood can be recognized by its bright red color and by the blood's spurting effect, which matches the rhythm of the pumping of the heart.

Venous bleeding is more easily controlled than arterial blood, and is a darker shade of red.

Capillary bleeding is the least serious. **Capillaries** are the blood vessels opened in minor cuts and grazes.

Severe bleeding

When a patient is bleeding heavily, soldiers will take immediate action to stop it. If the patient is bleeding from the veins or capillaries, then pressure is applied over the bleeding point. (Even minor arterial bleeding can be controlled with local pressure.) Troops will use anything to stop the blood flow, such as an item of clothing or a dressing. However, they are taught that it is important to try to make

Blood loss is a serious matter. This soldier makes medical notes after dressing the head wound of a simulated casualty.

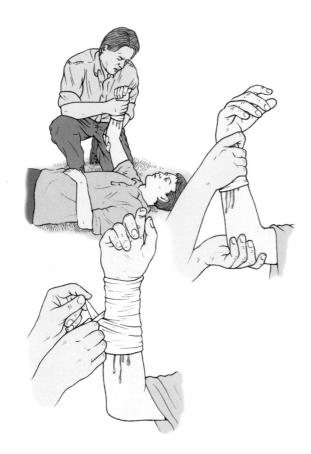

If the patient is bleeding from the veins or capillaries, pressure is applied over the bleeding point.

sure whatever they use is clean and **sterile**. Firm and continuous pressure is then maintained for around 5 to 10 minutes. Troops use a dressing to keep the wound clean.

Arterial bleeding

This is the most serious type of bleeding. Pressure on the major artery feeding an injured area will reduce or stop the flow of blood. The spots on the body where an artery can be easily compressed against a bone are called pressure points.

Pressure points for arterial bleeding are located in the:
- Temple, forward of ear
- Face, below eyes, side of jaw
- Shoulder or upper arm
- Elbow, underside of arm
- Lower arm, crook of elbow
- Hand, front of wrist
- Thigh, midway between the groin/top of knee

- Lower leg, upper side of knee
- Foot, front of ankle

Tourniquets

Elite troops use these only when severe bleeding cannot be controlled by any other method. **Tourniquets** can be placed only on the upper arm (just below the armpit) and around the upper thigh. Elite soldiers use a cloth at least two inches wide. They wrap the cloth around the limb and tie a half-knot. A stick is then placed over the knot and a double knot is tied over this. The stick is then twisted to tighten the tourniquet until the bleeding stops.

Warning—the loosening of a tourniquet can cause severe shock leading to death. (**Toxins** build up in the injured limb and then flood the heart when released.) If a tourniquet is applied, troops are aware that the limb may eventually be **amputated**.

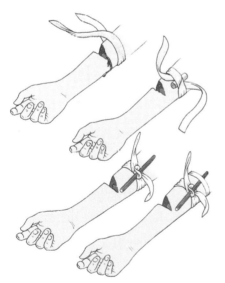

Use tourniquets only in the case of severe bleeding, tied around the upper arm or thigh.

Effects of blood loss

- One pint (475 ml). A person who loses this amount of blood may feel a little **faint** (as long as their vital organs, such as lungs and liver, are not affected).
- Two pints (1 liter). To lose this amount is more serious and the body starts to respond

to a more serious challenge. The casualty's blood pressure will begin to drop. This means that the body may not get enough oxygen. The person may become very faint, pale, and wobbly on the feet.

• Four pints (1.9 liters). With this much blood loss, the casualty can collapse. They will have a rapid, weak pulse. The skin will become clammy and pale as blood is diverted to major organs. The casualty may feel very sick and thirsty.

• Six pints (2.8 liters). With this much blood loss, the situation becomes life-threatening. The casualty will probably be unconscious; cardiac arrest and respiratory failure can soon follow.

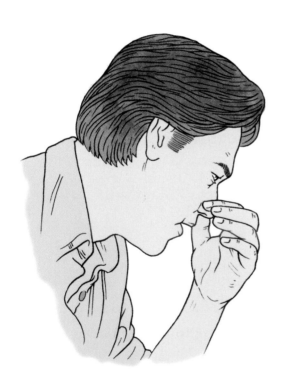

The best means of controlling a nosebleed is to lean forward and pinch the nostrils.

Internal bleeding

This results after a violent blow, broken bones, or deep wounds. Internal bleeding is indicated by faintness, light-headedness, pale skin that is cold and clammy to touch, red-colored urine, blood passed with feces, vomiting blood, and coughing blood.

To treat, an elite soldier will lay the patient flat on the back with the legs elevated. The patient will then be kept warm while waiting for rescue.

Wounds

Soldiers "irrigate" wounds with sterile **saline** solution or clean water. This means they wash it by pouring or squirting, not scrubbing. Butterfly bandages are used if the wound is not too deep. This is where the soldier's medical kit comes in useful, as the wound should be coated lightly with an antibiotic **ointment** before a sterile dressing and bandage is put on.

Nosebleeds

A nosebleed is a simple and common cause of blood loss, which can be caused by even the mildest knock. The patient is seated with the head slightly forward, and told to pinch the nostrils while breathing through the mouth. Sniffing is discouraged because this can let blood be swallowed and induce vomiting. Once bleeding is stopped, the patient is told not to touch or rub the nose for several hours, since this may restart the bleeding. If the bleeding persists for more than 30 minutes, then further help is required.

Bleeding from the ear

Bleeding from the ear should be taken very seriously. It can be a sign of brain damage. This will be indicated by a leakage of a thin, watery diluted blood. Other causes include a burst eardrum or something stuck inside the ear. In this case, blood will have a more regular texture and color. A soldier's treatment of ear bleeding begins with placing the patient in the recovery position. The bleeding ear should be angled downward to encourage drainage. The ear should be covered with a light sterile dressing and bandage.

Bleeding from the mouth

Bleeding from the mouth is usually caused by either a direct impact to the mouth, which bursts a lip, knocks out a tooth, or damages the gums, or by the teeth clamping onto the lip, gum, or tongue through an impact to the jaw. Either way, the bleeding can become serious.

If the injury is to the lip, an elite soldier pinches the wound between a pad and a finger. About 10 minutes of this pressure should stop the bleeding. No attempt is made to rinse the mouth out with water because this may restart the bleeding.

Burns

Burns can be life-threatening in a survival situation. There are three types of burns:

- First degree, which usually involve the first layer of skin. Not serious.
- Second degree, which involves the second layer of skin. These burns are very red, produce blisters, and are intensely painful for up to 48 hours. There is fluid loss and a danger of infection.
- Third degree, which destroys the first two layers of skin and damages deeper tissues. There is severe fluid loss and a danger of infection. The burned area is usually black, and the victim will suffer great pain.

Troops will make someone suffering from burns drink lots of water. The elite forces are also always prepared to treat burn victims for shock.

Military units have to deal with explosives and munitions, which can cause horrific burns. Here is how Canada's elite deal with them:

- They wash the burn immediately with cool water.
- They wash with peroxide followed by a light coating of iodine. Then they coat with an antibiotic ointment.
- They cover with a sterile bandage but do not use an airtight dressing.
- They remove the dressing every day and scrub the wound with a sterile gauze pad and peroxide.
- All white and yellow dead tissue is removed every day.
- They repeat the cleansing and dressing process.

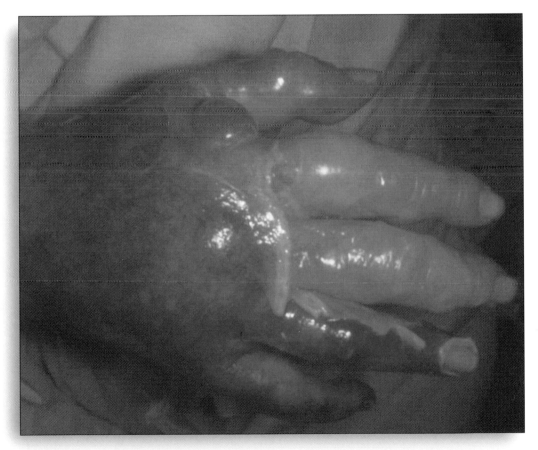

Burns are a common phenomenon in chemical warfare and can be life-threatening. This is an example of a third-degree burn.

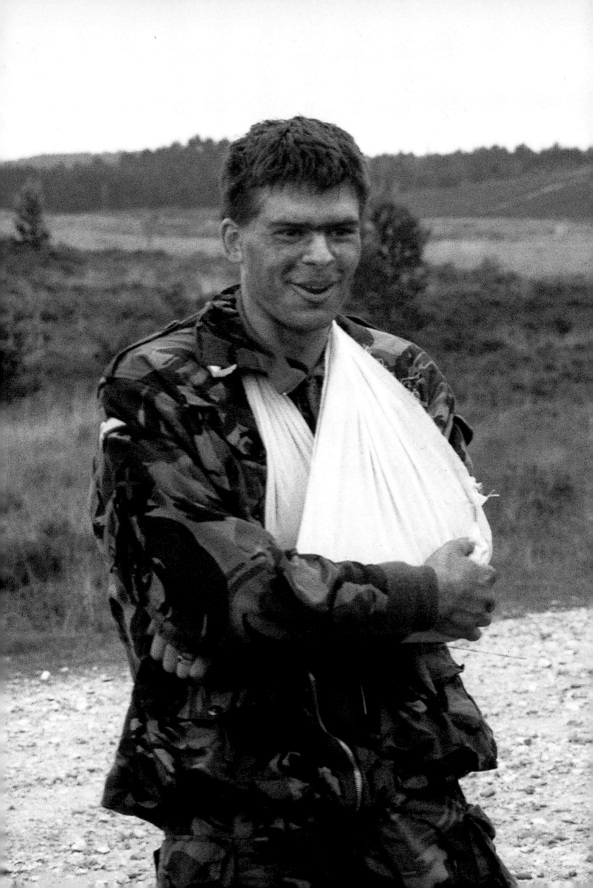

BONE, JOINT, AND MUSCLE INJURIES

Since the work of the elite forces can involve much physical activity, they are particularly prone to bone breakages and muscle injuries. This chapter demonstrates the first-aid treatments they use to cope with this when out in the field.

Breaks and fractures

A fracture is a chip, crack, or break of a bone. There are two types of fracture: open and closed. With an open fracture, the bone has come through the skin or something has penetrated the skin and then broken the bone. With a closed fracture, the bone is broken but there is no opening of the skin.

A fractured limb is **splinted** in exactly the same position that it is found in to prevent it from being damaged further while the patient is being taken to a hospital. Padding is used to keep the limb in position.

The Special Forces are experts in survival medicine. Use their training and identify the symptoms that can indicate a fractured limb.

- Patient feels or hears the bone break.
- Partial or complete loss of motion.
- Grating sound when limbs are moved.
- If the bone looks out of place, for example, or if the arm is bending but not at the elbow.

For soldiers, bone fractures are commonplace. One of the most basic first-aid lessons they learn is how to put an arm in a sling.

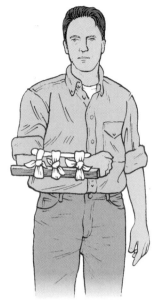

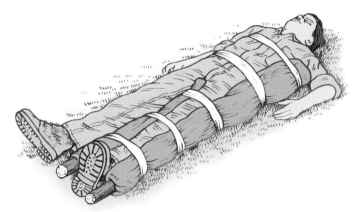

A splint—which can be made from sticks, branches, or boards—is used to prevent any further damage to a broken or fractured bone.

• Tenderness around the injury.
• Muscle spasm.

Closed fracture

If the casualty has a suspected closed fracture, then his or her pulse is checked at the wrist. If **circulation** is impeded (the hands feel cold or there is no pulse), it is important for the soldier to restore the flow of blood to the lower arm at once; otherwise the limb will have to be amputated.

The casualty's hand is pinched or poked to check and see if he or she feels anything. A member of the elite forces knows it is very serious if the patient has no feeling. **Traction** (a continuous pull) is then applied to try to restore some pulse and nerve response.

It is not a major concern if the casualty has only a little feeling. In fact, it means that the casualty can wait to be back in civilization for complete restoration. Full nerve response can often be restored by surgical techniques, and a trained soldier will reassure the patient of this.

If the patient has some feeling, a splint is securely applied. The joint should be immobilized on either side of the fracture.

Open fracture

- First, it is important for the elite soldier to control the bleeding if it is severe.
- The wound and the bone sticking out are then cleaned. The soldier then gives traction and tries to reset the fracture and close the wound. This is done slowly.
- After traction, the wound is inspected to ensure the bone ends join properly.

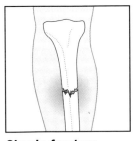
Simple fracture

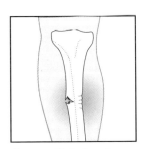
Greenstick fracture

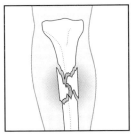
Comminuted fracture

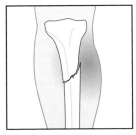
Closed fracture

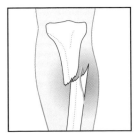
Open fracture

Diagrams showing differing types of fracture. The treatment given to a patient will vary depending on the seriousness of the break.

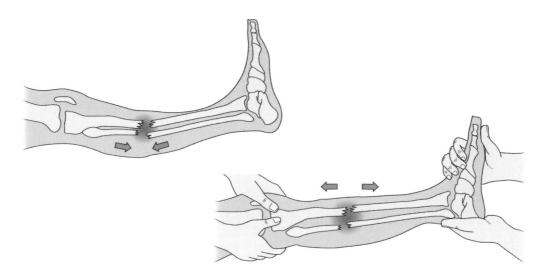

Traction (a continuous pull) is required to reposition a bone in its normal position. It should also restore some pulse and nerve response.

• The soldier then applies a splint, but in a way that leaves the wound free for treatment.

Throughout this time, the patient's pulse and nerve response will be checked. If any are missing, then the soldier needs to repeat the resetting and traction procedures.

Fractured ribs

For fracture of the upper ribs, patients are told to hold their breath while two long adhesive strips are applied across the shoulder of the injured side. For fracture of the lower ribs, a piece of felt or foam rubber is applied over the fracture.

Fractures take four to six weeks to heal. Fractured ribs can be painful; it is therefore important for the patient to get as much rest as possible.

Skull fracture

Indications of a fractured skull can be straw-colored fluid seeping from the ear or nose. If this occurs, patients are placed in the recovery position, with the leaking side down. Fluid is then able to escape, and patients are told not to move but to make themselves comfortable.

Neck fracture

Movement in a patient's neck can be stopped using a cervical collar, or by placing a small rolled towel or sheet under the neck and then placing sandbags or boots filled with dirt or sand on either side of the head to stabilize it. The patient should not move until rescued.

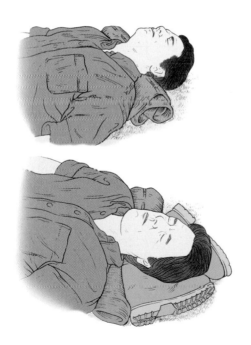

A patient with a neck fracture must be stabilized as soon as possible.

Breaks

In survival situations, it is usually toes and fingers that are broken. A soldier will reset the finger and then splint it with wood or something similar. Broken toes can be reset and taped to an unbroken toe next to it.

Spinal injuries

Any injury to the **spinal** column can cause paralysis and is potentially fatal. Signs of spinal injury include: a pain in the back

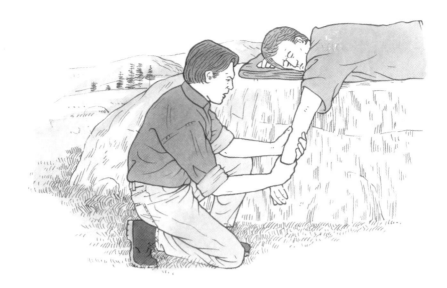

Traction being applied on a dislocated shoulder. The position of the casualty makes it easier for the attendant to perform the task.

without movement; any spot along the spinal column tender to the touch; loss of bladder control.

Spinal injuries are extremely dangerous. Always be careful when attempting to move a patient with a spinal injury.

- If the patient is faceup, a folded blanket is placed under the small of the back to stop pieces of bone cutting or pressing into the spine.
- If the patient is facedown, a folded blanket is placed under the chest.
- The back is always kept straight.

Strains, sprains, and dislocations

All of these can be common in a survival situation. A strain is a tearing or overstretching of a muscle. A sprain is a wrenching or tearing of tissues connected with the joint. A dislocation is usually caused by a fall, blow, or sudden force applied to a joint. This forces the joint out of place.

For strains, a soldier will rest the limb and apply cold packs to ease the pain. It is important to do this straight after injury, in order to reduce the swelling and pain.

British Special Air Service (SAS) soldiers fight on foot most of the time, and can suffer sprained ankles. They therefore have to have effective treatments for sprains.
• Bathe sprain with cold water to reduce swelling.
• Support with a bandage; do not constrict circulation.
• Raise affected limb and rest completely.

If you sprain an ankle, keep your boot on if you have to keep walking: the boot will act as a splint. If you take it off, the swelling will prevent you from putting it back on again.

Dislocations
When dislocations occur, swelling begins and the injury will be very sore. The joint must be reset before the swelling and muscle spasms begin; otherwise resetting will be difficult. The muscles near the joint will start to tighten up almost immediately. If this is not done, it may result in the casualty getting **gangrene** or other problems.

The two most important things a member of the elite forces is trained to remember about resetting a joint is to do it properly and do it as soon as possible.

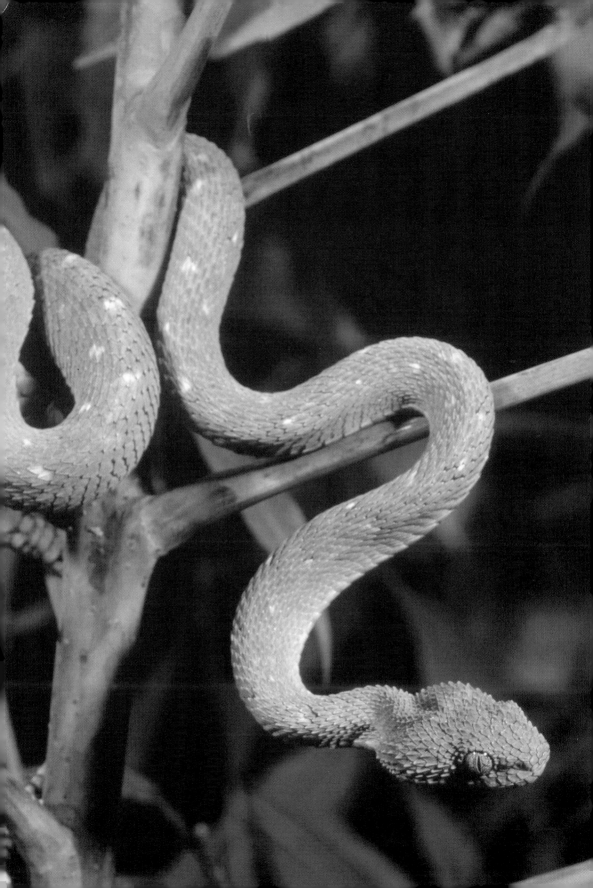

POISONS AND BITES

Poisoning and bites by spiders, centipedes, scorpions, and ants can be very painful and can make a person sick and possibly even die, so troops always learn what creatures live in the area where they are operating. To treat a bite from a scorpion or spider, the wound is cleaned and the poison is removed by suction or squeezing the bite. If soldiers have tobacco, they are trained to chew it and place it over the bite area. This will ease the pain. They treat the bite in the same way they would treat an open wound.

Because its soldiers often have to fight in regions where there is a lot of insect life, the U.S. Army has created some very effective anti-insect measures. They do not underestimate the danger of insects. Here are some guidelines given to U.S. troops:

- Inspect your body at least once a day to ensure there are no insects attached to you.
- Cover any ticks with Vaseline, heavy oil, or tree sap to cut off their air supply. The tick will release its hold and you can remove it. (Grasp it where the mouth parts are attached to the skin.) Wash your hands afterward and clean the tick wound thoroughly each day.
- Wash your skin well with soap and water if you have been in a mite-infested area.

The South-East Asian Greenbush viper is one of the most poisonous snakes in the world. If bitten, the soldier can die within 24 to 48 hours.

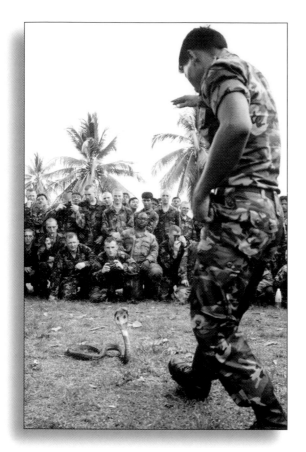

During jungle survival training, a Thai soldier demonstrates to his class how to handle a cobra.

• If stung by a bee or wasp, immediately remove the stinger and **venom** sac by scraping with a fingernail or knife. Do not squeeze it. Wash the wound thoroughly with soap and water and apply an ice pack or compress.

Relieve itching caused by insect bites by applying cold compresses, a cooling paste of mud and ashes, dandelion sap, coconut meat, or crushed leaves of garlic.

Snake bites

The chances of being bitten by a venomous snake in a survival situation are small. Nevertheless, it can happen and members of the elite forces must know how to treat snake bites.

Snakes are split into a number of types:
• Crotalidae—pit vipers.
• Elapidae—coral snakes, kraits, cobras, mambas, and asps.
• Hydrophine—sea snakes.
• Colubridae—backfanged boomslang.

Symptoms of snake bite

With the crotalidae bite there will be swelling at the bite site, which will slowly spread to the surrounding area. Swelling begins within three minutes and may continue for an hour. There is severe pain at the bite site and fang marks. Another symptom is blood in the urine. The venom will gradually destroy organs and blood cells. The victim will suffer severe headaches and thirst, a fall in blood pressure, and a corresponding rise of pulse rate, and bleeding into surrounding tissues. There is a real danger of a loss of limbs, and death can occur within 24 to 48 hours if the bite is serious and left untreated. (Vipers account for the majority of snake bite fatalities throughout the world.)

The elapidae and colubridae type of bite cause irregular heartbeat, a drop in blood pressure, weakness and **exhaustion**, severe headaches, dizziness, blurred vision, confusion, loss of muscular control, breathing difficulties, tingling, excessive **perspiration**, numbness of the lips and soles of the feet, chills, nausea, diarrhea, and loss of consciousness.

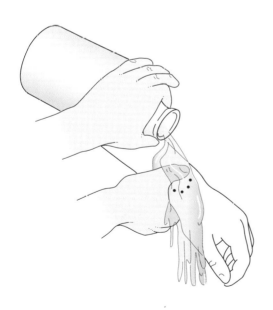

The hydrophine bite is usually painless. However, a bite should be suspected one to two hours after the onset of muscular aches, pains, and stiffness. The casualty will

Poisonous bites must be washed thoroughly with clean water. An ice pack will slow the spread of poison.

have reddish-brown urine within three hours. Death usually occurs within 12 to 24 hours without treatment.

All snake-bite victims will need treatment for shock. If no antivenom is available, then a restricting bandage, not a tourniquet, should be placed above the bite. Cold water or ice is used to keep the bite area as cool as possible.

U.S. Special Forces' tips—snake bite treatment

The Special Forces use the following treatment for snake bites in the wild:

• Kill the snake if you are the one bitten: it will make snake identification easier.

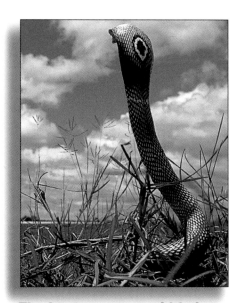

The best way to avoid being bitten by a snake is to stay out of its way. Most snakes attack only when provoked.

• Lie the patient down and make sure he or she does not move the injured part.
• Keep the patient warm and quiet.
• Begin specific treatment for snake types:

Crotalidae
• Make a clean cut about a quarter inch (5 mm) deep along, or in the direction of, the muscles through the puncture site. Do not make an X-cut and do not cut into joints.
• Apply suction using a mechanical

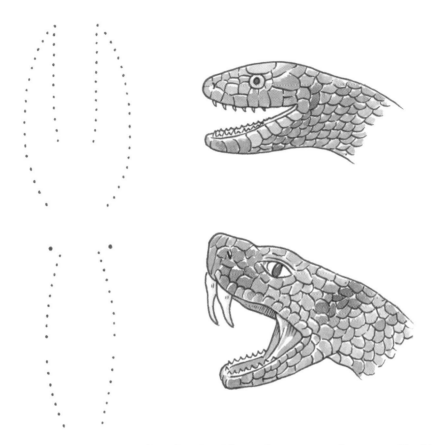

Not all snakes are harmful. Snake bites that are poisonous (bottom) and nonpoisonous (top) can be identified by the pattern of the bite.

device. (Do not use your mouth; you risk spreading the poison and are also unlikely to be able to extract much poison from the bite.) Suction should not be used if antivenom can be given within one hour or if it is over one hour since the bite.

• Do not use a tourniquet, tight bandages, or cold packs.

• Do not let the patient eat food or drink alcohol.

• Give patient small amounts of water at frequent intervals.

• Inject antivenom.

• Use morphine or other suitable painkillers as necessary.

Elapidae and colubridae

• Apply a tourniquet around the affected limb over a single bone (above the knee or below the lbow), which should be tight enough to stop arterial flow. It should be released for 30 seconds every 20 minutes to let fresh blood into the affected area.

• Inject antivenom.

Note: Do not administer morphine or other drugs that cause respiratory depression.

Hydrophine

Antivenom is the only treatment for hydrophine snake types. Incision and suction are of no value.

TREATMENT FOR POISONING—BRITISH SAS

SAS soldiers have fought all over the world for over 50 years. They have well-tested rules for dealing with poisons.

• In the case of suspected plant poisoning, elite troops make the person vomit. Alternatively, they make an antidote by mixing tea and charcoal with an equal part of milk of magnesia if available. The charcoal absorbs the poison and carries it from the body.

• They then wash the poisoned skin with soap and water. With inhaled poisons, they move the patient into a place that has fresh air, loosen tight clothing, and give artificial respiration.

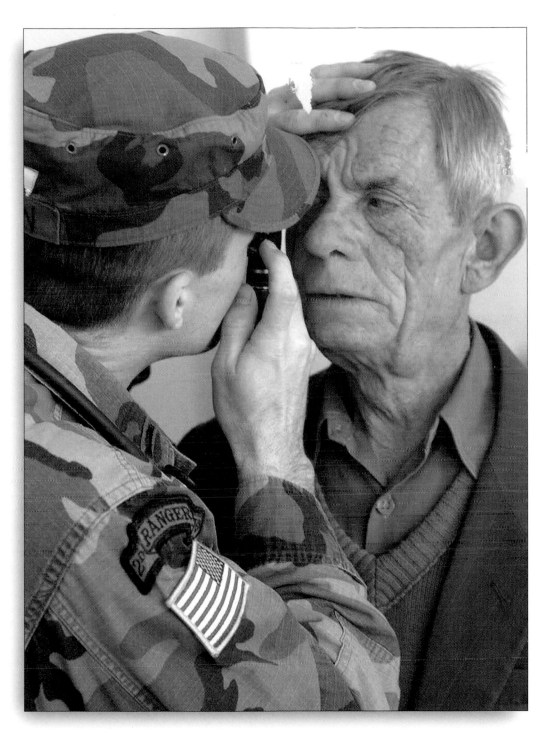

Treatment is required immediately if the eyes come into contact with animal poison. If it is not received, the victim can easily be blinded.

GLOSSARY

Abdominal Relating to the stomach area.

Amputated To sever a limb, usually if it is seriously infected.

Antiseptic Cream/lotion that fights infection.

Artery A major blood vessel.

Cardiac Having to do with the heart.

Casualty An injured person.

Capillaries Small veins.

Circulation Blood flow.

Compression Pushing together.

Dislocations Joints out of place.

Exhaustion Tiredness.

Faint To lose consciousness.

Fracture Chip, crack, or break.

Gangrene Rotting of the flesh as a result of a wound.

Hypodermic Injecting needle.

Hypothermia Serious condition caused by extreme cold.

Ointment Lotion.

Perspiration Sweat.

Pulse Beat of the heart, which sends blood around the body.

Puritabs Tablets that release chlorine to clean water and make it drinkable.

Recovery position A common position in which to place casualties, on their side.

Respiration Breathing.

Resuscitation Process of helping a person to breathe.

Saline Containing and/or tasting of salt.

Spasm Sudden uncontrolled movement.

Spinal Connected with the backbone.

Splinted Held in place rigidly with a stick or other stiff object.

Sterile Germ-free.

Symptoms Signs of disease or injury.

Thermometer Device used to measure the temperature of a person.

Tourniquets Tight bandages to restrict the flow of blood.

Toxins Poisons.

Traction A continuous pull.

Venom Snake or other animal poison.

EQUIPMENT REQUIREMENTS

Basic Medical Pack
Thermometer—to check a patient's temperature
Gudel airway—to help maintain an open airway when someone is unconscious
Gauze—disinfected material for dressing wounds
Paraffin gauze dressing—see above
Scalpel blades (at least two)
Suture equipment—to stitch up wounds
Large safety pins
Scissors
Antiseptic swabs—to prevent infection
Green hypodermic needles—used for removing splinters and for draining blisters
Fluid-replacement packets—used for people suffering from diarrhea and burns
Puritabs—releases chlorine to clean water and make it drinkable
Potassium permanganate—used as an antifungal/disinfectant
Painkillers
Antacid tablets—used for indigestion.
Antidiarrhea tablets
Antihistamine tablets—for bites and allergies
Plasters and wound dressings
Sunblock and lip balm

Clothing and shelter
Thermal underwear
Thin layer of synthetic material
Woolen or wool mixture shirt
Woven fiber sweater or jacket (normally a fleece)
Waterproof and windproof final layer
Two pairs of socks (minimum)
Compact, light, windproof pants with numerous pockets with zippers, to carry
    items securely.
Waterproof pants
Gloves—leather or mittens
Balaclava (a tight woolen garment covering the head and neck, except for parts of
    the face)
Spare clothing—socks, underwear, shirts, etc.
Soft, well-maintained leather boots
H-frame backpack with side pockets
Portable, lightweight, waterproof shelter

Survival bag
Pliers with wire cutter
Dental floss (for sewing)
Folding knife
Ring saw
Snow shovel
Signal cloth
Fishing hooks and flies
Weights and line
Multivitamins
Protein tablets
Large chocolate bar
Dried eggs
Dried milk

File
Cutlery set
Three space blankets
Four candles
Microlite flashlight
Extra battery and bulb
Fire starter
Windproof and waterproof matches
Butane lighter
Insect repellent
Snares
Plastic cup
Slingshot and ammunition
Knife sharpener

USEFUL WEBSITES

http://depts.washington.edu/learncpr/index.html
http://www.medicinenet.com
http://library.thinkquest.org/10624/index.html
http://www.clark.net/pub/electra/cse0.html
http://www.princeton.edu/oa/safety/wildsafe.html
http://www.redcross.org
http://www.cdc.gov/niosh/nasd/docs3/me97010.html

FURTHER READING

Craig, Glen. *US Army Special Forces Medical Handbook*. London: Paladin, 1998.

Darman, Peter. *The Survival Handbook*. London: Greenhill Books, 1996.

Department of Army. *First Aid for Soldiers*. New York: Apple Pie Publishers, 1999

Gill, Paul. *The Onboard Medical Guide*. Rockport, Me.: International Marine Publishing, 1996.

Laffin, John. *Combat Surgeons*. Gloucester, England: Sutton Publishing, 1999.

McNab, Chris. *First Aid Survival Manual*. Edison, N.J.: Book Sales, 2001.

Mears, Ray. *The Outdoor Survival Handbook*. London: Ebury Press, 2001.

ABOUT THE AUTHOR

Patrick Wilson was educated at Marlborough College, Wiltshire and studied history at Manchester University. He was a member of the Officer Training Corps, and for the past seven years he has been heavily involved in training young people in the art of survival on Combined Cadet Force (CCF) and Duke of Edinburgh Courses. He has taught history at St. Edward's School, Oxford, Millfield School, and currently at Bradfield College in England.

His main passion is military history. His first book was *Dunkirk—From Disaster to Deliverance* (Pen & Sword, 2000). Since then he has written *The War Behind the Wire* (Pen & Sword, 2000), which accompanied a television documentary on prisoners of war. He recently edited the diaries of an Australian teenager in the First World War.

INDEX

References in italics refer to illustrations

ABC method of assessment 15–18
airways, checking 15–16
arterial bleeding 37, 38–39
artificial respiration 23–24
artificial resuscitation 17, 23–27
assessing the situation 14–21

bites 53–59
bleeding 37–42
    on the head 18
    open fractures 47
blisters 9
blocked airways 29–30
blood loss, effects of 39–40
bone injuries 44–51
breathing, checking 16–17, 19, 20, 23–33
burns 42–43

capillary bleeding 37
carbon monoxide poisoning 31
cardiac massage 25–26
cardiopulmonary resuscitation (CPR) 23, 26–27
casualty drills 6, 8, 13
checking a pulse 17–18
chemical warfare 43
chest, listening for breathing 19
Chilean Air Force CPR 26
choking 29–30
circulation 17–18, 33–35
    after bone fractures 46
closed fractures 46–47
clothing 61
colubridae snake bites 55, 58
course of action 14–21
CPR (cardiopulmonary resuscitation) 23, 26–27
crotalidae snake bites 55, 56–57

dangers in emergency situations

assessing the risk of 13
    from smoke or gas 32
DATE system 13
dental problems 9
diagnosis 13, 18–21
dislocations 50, 51
    of the jaw 19
drowning accidents 27–29

ears, bleeding from 41
elapidae snake bites 55, 58
emergency drills 6, 8, 13
emergency situations
    assessment 13
    dangers in 13, 32
    diagnosis 13, 18–21
    preparation 9–11
equipment requirements 9–11, 61–62
evacuation 13
    by helicopter 14
eyes
    animal poison in 59
    examining 19

feet
    breaking bones in toes 49
    checking for spinal damage 20–21
finger breaks 49
first aid kits 10, 11, 61
fractured ribs 48–49
fractures, bone 45–50
French Foreign Legion
    cardiac massage 25–26
fume inhalation 31–32

glossary 60

hands
    examining 20
    finger breaks 49
head, skull fracture 49
head-to-toe diagnosis 18–21
heart massage 25–26
Heimlich Maneuver 31
helicopters, for evacuation 14
hydrophine snake bites

55–56, 58
hypothermia 29, 34–35

inhaled poisons 58
injections 9–10
insects, dangerous 53–54
internal bleeding 40
internet addresses 62

jabs 9–10
jaw, dislocations of 19
joint injuries 44–51
jungle survival training 54

legs, checking for spinal damage 20–21

medical packs 10, 11, 61
mouth
    bleeding from 42
    checking for injuries 19
mouth-to-mouth respiration 23–24
muscle injuries 50–51

near-drowning 27–29
neck
    examining 19
    fractures 49
nosebleeds 41, 41

open fractures 47–48

plant poisoning 58
poisons 53–59
preparation 9–11
pressure points, to stop bleeding 38–39
pulse, checking 17–18

rapid assessment 15–18
recovery position 16
resuscitation, artificial 17, 23–27
ribs, fractured 48–49
Royal Thai Marines
    casualty drills 8

saline solutions 41
SAS (British)
    first aid kits 11
    gas masks 32

poisoning, treatment for 58
sprained ankles 51
shelter 61
shock 33–35
    after snake bites 56
    following burns 42
skin, changes in color 19, 20
skull fractures 49
smoke inhalation 31–32
snake bites 52, 54–59
spinal injuries 49–50
splinting fractures 45, 46
sprains and strains 50–51
survival bag 62

taking a pulse 17–18
talking to the injured 14
teamwork 15
teeth 9
toes, breaking 49
tourniquets 39–40
traction, to straighten bones 46, 48, 50

U.S. Army
    anti-insect measures 53–54
U.S. Marine Corps
    cardiac massage 25–26
    decontamination exercise 33
    first aid kits 11
    keeping the injured calm 14
U.S. Navy SEALs
    training program 28
U.S. Special Forces
    first aid kits 11
    snake bites 56–58

vaccinations 9–10
venous bleeding 37

web sites 62
wounds 37–42